80 Homemade Natural Hair Care and Hair Growth Recipes

Hair Loss Treatment and Hair Growth Remedies (Natural Hair Care

Recipes for Hair Health and Hair Growth)

MATILDA C BUTLER

DEDICATION

To all who desire to live life to the fullest!

TABLE OF CONTENT

INTRODUCTION

Do you know you can make your own beauty products like shampoo, hair conditioner, detangler and so on from the comfort of your own home? Yea maybe not! You probably never thought of it. With the alarming number of store bought cosmetics and beauty products available in the market, it would be difficult to think of anyone taking the time to make DIY beauty and hair products for the personal beauty routine. Well there are numerous advantages to making your own hair care products at home, and I will be explaining some of these advantages below.

a) Its purse friendly; and you cut extra cost.

Just like several other items, homemade hair care products are super cheap compared to store-bought commercial made hair care products. Putting numbers into consideration; making your own hair care products is the best option for you, if you have a large family like mine.

b) Your health is wealth.

Several toxic and hazardous chemicals go into the production and packaging of synthetic hair care products, even when "natural", "all-natural" is written on the label. Adequate regulations are not put in place to properly regulate, check mate and ensure the safety of most beauty care products we buy and use. Big beauty care and cosmetic producing companies like Suave and Aussie, Pantene among several others use chemicals that are known to cause immunotoxicity, allergies, cancer, and the likes. Needless to say, making your own beauty products and hair care products is the safe way to go, to ensure the safety of the ingredients used and to avoid damage to health on the long term.

c) Efficiency.

So many cosmetics, beauty and hair products make unrealistic promises that never get fulfilled. Making your own beauty and hair products gives you the power and flexibility to create things that would work for you perfectly, your hair type, color and texture.

This is somehow very subjective; but a greater percentage of people say that they have had more results with homemade hair products than store bought commercial brands.

d) Environmental Health.

When you make your own hair care products, you are in charge and your ingredients are natural and organic. Store bought commercial shampoos, conditioner, detanglers and so on contain several tons of harmful chemicals. When natural hair products go down the drain, the environment is safe compared to the synthetic hair products which poisons our water system on the long run.

e) Home Health.

Natural ingredients are safer for your house pipes; they do not damage your pipelines or cause pipeline damage over a period of time. This safety should be put into consideration when considered which hair and beauty products to go for.

CHAPTER ONE- ORGANIC DIY SHAMPOO HAIR TREATMENT

You can make your own shampoo and give your hair the care, treatment and pampering it deserves.

Castile Flavored Shampoo

Ingredients

¼ cup liquid Castile soap

¼ cup water

½ tsp oil (like grapeseed, olive oil or jojoba)

Instructions

1. Combine Liquid castile soap, water and any oil of your choice.

2. Mix together and combine well.

3. Transfer mixture into a plastic or glass bottle.

4. Shake well before each use.

NOTE: This combination works well for some hair types, textures and colors. For some others, they have reported that the shampoo leaves a film on their hair. The type of hair you have and the type of water used can have so much impact on the result gotten from this shampoo's use.

Simple Shampoo for Your Hair

This shampoo gives a really impressive lather.

Ingredients

Foaming Bottles or Flip Cap Bottles to dispense

¼ cup of liquid Castile Soap (unscented or your favorite)

¼ cup of water (distilled)

½ tsp of grapeseed, jojoba or other light vegetable oil

Instructions

1. Combine Liquid castile soap, water and any oil of your choice.

2. Mix together and combine well.

3. Transfer mixture into a flip cap bottle.

4. Shake well before each use.

5. Apply by tilting the bottle slightly over your head.

Baking Soda with Apple Cider Vinegar Shampoo

Ingredients

3 cups water

1/2 cup baking soda

1/2 cup apple cider vinegar/ regular white vinegar

Instructions

1. Combine baking soda and warm water together.

2. Stir to combine until thoroughly mixed.

3. Transfer into a plastic or glass container.

4. Shake well before each use.

5. Apply by scrubbing shampoo into your scalp.

6. Wash off with vinegar.

TIP: You may decide to tweak ingredient ratios slightly until you find what works for you perfectly.

NOTE: It takes 2-4 weeks for your body to adjust to this new shampoo. Before now, you probably have been using store bought commercial products which have stripped your body of natural oils on a daily basis. Once you start using this natural shampoo, you hair may start to feel thick or oily as you start to gradually adjust.

Hair Waking Shampoo

At some point you may want to stimulate and wake up your scalp from its sleep. The ingredients in this recipe will help make that a reality.

Ingredients

1/8 teaspoon tea tree essential oil

¼ cup water (distilled)

1/8 teaspoon peppermint essential oil

2 teaspoon jojoba oil

¼ cup liquid Castile Soap (unscented or your favorite)

Flip Cap Bottles or Foaming Bottles to dispense

Instructions

1. Combine liquid castile soap with jojoba oil together in a small mixing bowl.

2. Stir together until well combined.

3. Add the distilled water and stir well.

4. Measure in tea tree and peppermint essential oils.

5. Stir well until oils have been well distributed.

6. Transfer mixture into a flip cap bottle.

7. Shake well before each use.

8. Apply as you would any regular shampoo.

9. Wash your hair and pat dry.

Easy to make Aromatherapy Shampoo Recipe

Ingredients

7 fluid ounces Unscented Shampoo Base

40 drops Lavender essential Oil

1 tbsp Jojoba {if desired} (gives the hair added hydration)

5 drops Ylang Ylang essential Oil

10 drops Rosemary essential Oil

Instructions

1. Get a mixing bowl,

2. Toss in the unscented shampoo base into the bowl,

3. Blend in lavender, jojoba, ylang ylang and rosemary essential oils.

4. Combine thoroughly until essential oils are well incorporated.

5. Pour shampoo into an 8 ounce bottle, using a funnel.

NOTE: Adhere to all essential oil safety precautions when using any essential oil or blend. Always do a skin patch test for essential oils before usage, make sure the essential oils you are using are gentle to the skin.

6. Apply as you would a regular shampoo.

Essential Aloe Vera Shampoo

This recipe is a hair growth potion that is anti-fungal and anti-bacterial.

Ingredients

1/4-1/2 cup water

Aloe Vera gel (better if it's fresh)

Rosemary essential oil

Instructions

1. Combine aloe gel, water and essential oil together in a bowl.

2. Stir together and transfer into an electric blender.

3. Blend until a smooth consistency has been reached.

4. Transfer mixture into a container.

Lavender Hair Care Shampoo

Ingredients

1 ½ tbsps of glycerin

1 cup castille soap (Lavender)

1 cup of water, distilled

6 chamomile tea bags

Instructions

1. Brew a cup of chamomile tea. Bring water to boiling.

2. Transfer into a tea cup and leave chamomile tea bags in the cup for 20 minutes.

3. Measure in liquid castile soap into the tea, stirring to combine.

4. Measure in glycerin into the tea mixture and stir thoroughly until well incorporated.

5. Transfer mixture into a dark glass bottle and cover well.

6. Store in a cool, dry and dark place.

Hair Drying Shampoo

Ingredients

¼ cup of distilled water

¼ cup of aloe vera gel

¼ cup of liquid Castile Soap (your favorite scent)

¼ tsp of jojoba oil or avocado oil

1 tsp of glycerin

Flip Cap Bottles or Foaming Bottles to dispense

Instructions

1. Combine aloe vera gel, liquid castile soap, avocado/jojoba oil, water, and glycerin together in a small mixing bowl.

2. Stir to combine until thoroughly mixed.

3. Transfer into a flip cap bottle.

4. Shake well before each use.

5. Apply by scrubbing shampoo into your scalp.

Glowing Hair Rosemary Shampoo

This recipe brings a radiant liveliness to your hair. It is fragrant and would add the desired and needed shine to your hair.

Ingredients

2 tablespoons of rosemary, dried

¼ cup of water, distilled

¼ cup of liquid Castile Soap (use lemon)

¼ lemon essential oil

2 tablespoons sweet almond oil

Flip Cap Bottles or Foaming Bottles to dispense

Instructions

1. Bring water to boiling in a pot over medium high heat.

2. Measure in rosemary and then leave for a while to release flavor into hot water, until water becomes fragrant.

3. Using a mesh strainer or cheesecloth, strain water from leaves and set rosemary flavored water aside to cool.

4. After cooling, measure in the liquid castile soap, sweet almond oil and lemon essential oil.

5. Stir well to combine.

6. Transfer mixture into a flip cap bottle and store in a cool, dry place.

7. Apply as you would a regular shampoo.

Hair Flake-Fighting Shampoo

This shampoo is a flaky scalp remedy; it will give your scalp and hair the freshness you deserve.

Ingredients

¼ cup of water, distilled

1 tbsp of apple cider vinegar

¼ cup of liquid Castile Soap

½ tsp of grapeseed, jojoba, or other light vegetable oil

6 finely ground cloves

3 tbsps of apple juice

Flip Cap Bottles or Foaming Bottles to dispense

Instructions

1. Combine vinegar, castile soap, grapeseed oil, water, ground cloves and apple juice together in a mixing bowl.

2. Transfer mixture into an electric blender or small grinder.

3. Blend mixture together for 30 seconds.

4. Transfer mixture into flip cap bottles.

5. Warm water, and wet your hair before applying shampoo as you would a regular shampoo.

6. Wash your hair and pat dry.

7. Refrigerate remaining shampoo.

NOTE: It has a 3 day shelf life.

Lavender Hair Shampoo

Ingredients

1 teaspoon of baking soda

¼ cup of oatmeal

1 teaspoon of lavender or other fragrant herb, crushed

Instructions

1. Combine oatmeal, baking soda and crushed lavender together in a small mixing bowl.

2. Transfer oatmeal mixture into a small grinder or a mortar and pestle.

3. Grind oatmeal mixture until thoroughly ground.

4. Transfer into a container.

5. Apply by sprinkling mixture to cover your scalp.

6. Use your hands to rub in the mixture into your scalp for 5 minutes.

7. Brush mixture out after 5 minutes.

NOTE: You can tweak ingredients ratio and produce in larger quantities.

8. Transfer remaining recipe into a container and store in a cool, dry place.

Deliciously Scented Shampoo

The fragrance of this shampoo is out of this world and only meant for Queens.

Ingredients

¼ cup liquid Castile Soap (your favorite)

¼ cup of water, distilled

10 drops of coconut fragrance oil

2 teaspoon of jojoba oil

10 drops of vanilla essential oil

Flip Cap Bottles or Foaming Bottles to dispense

Instructions

1. Combine liquid castile soap, coconut fragrance oil, jojoba oil and water together in a mixing bowl.

2. Stir well until well combined.

3. Measure in vanilla essential oil.

4. Stir to incorporate essential oil into the mixture.

5. Transfer Shampoo mixture into a flip cap bottle.

6. Apply as you would a regular shampoo.

7. Wash hair off and pat dry.

CHAPTER TWO - ORGANIC DIY CONDITIONER TREATMENT

Making your hair treatment right from your home has advantages that cannot be under emphasized. This hair treatment is focused on your type, texture and probably color of hair without being exposed to chemicals and additives that are synthetic, hazardous and toxic. When you condition your hair, you protect it from various hair stressors like the heat styling and harsh temperatures, poor diet, hormone irregularities and many more. When you condition your hair; a protective shield is formed over the whole hair shaft and your hair is re-moisturized, these in turn reduces the breaking of your hair.

Hair Care Blends; Choosing Carrier Oils Considering Your Kind Of Hair

Your hair has specific and peculiar needs that should be met as you make and apply every organic conditioner recipe.

The information below would guide and help you to efficiently create the specific blend that will suit your hair type.

You are free to combine these oils in different ways. Make combinations of two ingredients or three or all the ingredients; whatever works for you.

a) Normal Hair Care Blends

Coconut, olive, jojoba Oils

b) Oily Hair Care Blends

Jojoba, grapeseed Oils

c) Dry/Damaged/Frizzy Hair Care Blends

Jojoba, castor, olive, coconut oils and Shea butter

d) Dandruff Fighting Hair Care Blends

Castor, avocado, sesame, olive, coconut oils

e) Thinning Hair Care Blends

Sweet almond, olive, castor, avocado, grapeseed oils

TIP: When blending oils together in the hair care blends, the percentage of avocado oil used should be 10% only; avocado oil a very difficult to wash/rinse waxy residue.

Herbal Infusion for Simple Herbal Hair Conditioner

This conditioner recipe improves the health of your hair and brightens and enhances your hair color; and should be used in place of the distilled water in the recipe below.

Blonde Hair Peel	Dried Calendula, Chamomile, Lemon
Dark Hair	Black Tea, Dried Rosemary, Cloves
Red Hair Bark	Dried Calendula, Hibiscus, Cinnamon
Gray Hair	Dried Sage, Rosemary, Thyme

Ingredients

1 tbsp each herb blend (check your type of hair above)

1/4 cup distilled water

Instructions

1. Combine three tablespoons of the herb blend that suits your hair type into a mixing bowl.

2. Measure in distilled water into the herb blend.

3. Transfer mixture to a pot.

4. Bring distilled water mixture to a boil over medium heat.

5. Take off from heat and set aside for 60 minutes, to release flavors.

6. Use a mesh strainer or cheesecloth to strain out the herbs and save the herbal infused liquid.

7. Use herbal infusion in the recipe below to substitute distilled water.

Note: The gray hair herbal infusion smell very "herbal", but it would give you great results over few weeks of daily usage. It is worth it all the way.

Simple Herbal Conditioner

Ingredients

½ cup of herbal infusion/distilled water

1 tsp of Carrier Oil (check table above, for type of hair)

1 tbsp of (8g) Emulsifying Wax

Essential Oils for type of hair

½ teaspoon of Vitamin E

5 drops of pure GSE

1 tsp of Vegetable Glycerin

Instructions

1. Combine glycerin, wax and oil together in a small bowl.

2. Stir until well combined.

3. Transfer into a glass jar, and place into a pot partly filled with water and melt over low heat.

4. Take off from heat when wax melts completely.

5. Measure in the vit. E and stir.

6. Meanwhile warm herbal infusion or distilled water in another pot or in a microwave until lukewarm.

NOTE: Step 6 is very important to the end results of your hair conditioner.

7. Pour lukewarm herbal infusion or water into the wax mixture in a slow and steady stream, using a whisk to continue stirring as you pour, until a thick, smooth and creamy consistency is reached.

8. Set mixture aside to cool.

NOTE: Mixture gets thicker as it becomes cooler.

9. Once mixture is cool, measure in pure GSE and essential oil blend.

10. Transfer mixture into 8 oz dark bottle with a good cover.

NOTE: Do not cover until mixture cools completely. As the mixture cools, shake bottle from time to time so that ingredients will not separate.

11. Keep in a dark, dry cool place.

NOTE: Decrease the carrier oil quantity and choose grapeseed oil (it happens to be light), if your hair turns out to be greasy.

Correcting Fly-away Hair Ends

Ingredients

2-3 drops Jojoba oil

Instructions

1. Pour oil on your palm.

2. Put your palms against the other and rub in circles slightly.

3. Run oiled hands over your hair to straighten out fly away and frizzy hair ends.

Homemade Herbal Rinse

This rinse balances the pH of your scalp, reduces the buildup of hair care products after hair conditioning. It gives your hair the shine it deserves and helps the manageability of your hair.

Importance of Herbal Rinse

1. Fights against and heals inflammation.

2. Heals chemical and synthetic hair treatments skin problems

3. Serves as a dandruff treatment.

4. Reduces hair grease.

Ingredients

Herbs (check table below)

2 cups distilled water

Dark glass container

Normal-Dry Hair: 3 tbsps dried chamomile, 3 tbsps lavender

Thinning Hair/Oily Hair/Dandruff: 3 tbsps dried peppermint, 3 tbsps rosemary.

Instructions

1. Combine herb blends and distilled water together into a mixing bowl.

2. Transfer into a pot and bring to a boil over medium high heat.

3. Take off heat and set aside for 60 minutes to release flavors.

4. Use a mesh strainer or cheesecloth to strain out herbs.

5. Transfer herbal hair rinse into a dark glass bottle.

6. Apply by gently rubbing the rinse into your hair and scalp with your hands.

7. Wash out and pat dry.

CHAPTER THREE - ORGANIC DIY DEEP CONDITIONER HAIR TREATMENT

Fruity hair conditioner

Ingredients

1 Cup of coconut milk

2 tablespoon of Mango Butter/Oil

¼ Cup of Honey

Instructions

1. Combine coconut milk, mango butter and honey together into a mixing bowl.

2. Stir to combine, until well combined.

3. Transfer to a pot over medium low heat, and warm slightly.

4. Apply to slightly damp and clean hair.

5. Wrap the treated hair for 30-60 minutes with a plastic shower cap.

6. Wash off and pat hair dry.

Egg/Mayonnaise Flavored Hair Conditioner

Ingredients

2 eggs, beaten

1 cup mayonnaise

1 tbsp olive oil

Instructions

1. Combine eggs, mayonnaise and olive oil together into a small bowl.

2. Whip mixture until well mixed and a thick creamy consistency is reached.

3. Rub into your hair thoroughly to dry and clean.

4. Cover your hair with a plastic cap.

5. Use a hand-held blow drier or hood drier to dry hair for 20 minutes.

6. Wash off, pat dry and apply shampoo to your hair.

Mayonnaise/Cinnamon Hair Conditioner

This recipe hydrates your hair and gives your hair the needed shine.

Ingredients

Cinnamon

Mayonnaise

Honey

2 eggs, beaten

Few drops milk

Instructions

1. Combine cinnamon, mayonnaise, honey, eggs and a few drops of milks together into a small mixing bowl.

2. Transfer mixture to a pot and place over medium low heat until slightly warmed.

3. Apply and leave in your for 30-60 minutes.

Mayonnaise Treat

This conditioner has so many moisturizing agents, proteins and other hair growing substances. It promotes the growth of hair and should also be used to deep-condition your lovely curls.

Ingredients

3 tablespoons Honey

4 drops of Peppermint Essential Oil

4 tablespoons of mayonnaise

EVOO

1 Egg, beaten

EVCO

4 drops of Rosemary Essential Oil

Instructions

1. Combine honey, mayonnaise, evoo, beaten egg and evco together in a small mixing bowl.

2. Mix thoroughly until well combined.

3. Measure in peppermint and rosemary essential oils.

4. Stir thoroughly until essential oils are evenly distributed in the mixture.

5. Shampoo your hair before applying mayonnaise deep conditioner treat.

6. Leave on for 60 minutes.

7. Wash off and pat dry.

Hair Glow Deep Conditioner

Ingredients

½ cup of any moisturizing conditioner as a base

1 tablespoon of honey

½ of an avocado

2 teaspoon of black Jamaican castor oil

1 tablespoon of mayonnaise

2 teaspoon of coconut oil

You can substitute the oils to fit your hairs likings!

Instructions

1. Combine moisturizing conditioner and avocado together in a small bowl.

2. Transfer into an electric blender and blend until a smooth consistency is reached.

3. Remove avocado mixture from blender.

4. Stir in honey, castor oil, mayonnaise and coconut oil into the avocado mixture.

5. Stir until well incorporated.

6. Apply to hair and leave for some minutes, covering your hair with a plastic cap.

7. Wash off and pat hair dry.

Hot Coconut Hair Treatment

Use on damaged or normal hair..

Ingredients

1 teaspoon of calendula oil

1 tablespoon of coconut oil

Instructions

1. Combine calendula oil and coconut oil in a small mixing bowl.

2. Transfer into a double boiler over medium low heat.

3. Heat calendula oil mixture until melted.

4. Take off heat and set aside to cool slightly.

5. Stir together and apply warm mixture to the hair.

6. Cover hair with a towel for 5 minutes.

7. Wash off with warm water and pat hair dry.

Light Cream Hair Conditioner

Ingredients

1/2 cups of coconut milk

2 tbsp of olive oil

1 to 2 cups of yogurt

2 eggs, beaten

Instructions

1. Combine oil and eggs together in a small mixing bowl.

2. Stir in coconut milk and just enough yogurts to reach desired level of conditioner's thickness.

3. Stir well until a rich creamy consistency is reached.

4. Apply hair conditioner and leave on for 30-60 minutes.

5. Cover your hair with a plastic cap.

6. Wash off and pat hair dry.

Aloe Vera Tea Mask

This deep conditioning mask works for any hair type, gives the hair shine and softens it.

Ingredients

Aloe Vera gel

Green Tea

Coconut oil

Rosemary

Fresh ginger

Your favorite Essential oil

Instructions

1. Brew a hot cup of green tea.

2. Measure in coconut oil, rosemary, ginger and aloe vera.

3. Stir together and return to heat.

4. Bring to a boil for 5 minutes before taking off heat.

5. Set aside to cool.

6. Strain out tea bags and transfer the aloe vera liquid into a bowl.

7. Measure in the essential oil and stir to distribute evenly.

8. Apply to your hair, covering your hair ends well, leave on for 60 minutes.

9. Wash hair with warm water and pat dry.

NOTE: If coconut oil doesn't suit your hair type, feel free to substitute another oil type.

Castornnaise Deep Conditioner

This recipe is designed for a 12 inches long hair or lesser; feel free to adjust ingredients for a longer hair length

Ingredients:

1 tbsp mayonnaise

1 egg, beaten

1 tsp cold pressed castor oil

1-2 tsps olive oil

1 drop vitamin E oil

1 tbsp rinse out conditioner, if desired

Instructions

1. Combine mayonnaise, beaten egg, castor oil, olive oil and vitamin E oil together in a small mixing bowl.

2. Stir thoroughly until well combined.

3. Wash hair well before application.

4. Apply to damp hair massaging into every part of your hair and scalp.

5. Wear plastic cap.

6. Leave on for 20-30 minutes before rinsing out.

TIP: Use rinse out conditioner when rinsing out.

Honey Glow Deep Conditioner Hair Treatment

Ingredients

Some cond. (Aussie Moist)

1 1/3 cup of honey

1 cup of Coconut oil

1 inch of olive oil

3 tbsps of Lemon Juice

Instructions

1. Combine all ingredients aside the oils together into a bowl.

2. Transfer coconut and olive oil into a glass bottle.

3. Place bottle in a pot partly filled with water, and warm over medium low heat for 2 minutes.

4. Wash your hair and pour mixture on your hair before pouring the coconut/olive oil mixture also.

5. Leave on and cover your hair with a plastic cap for 30 minutes.

CHAPTER FOUR - ORGANIC HAIR DETANGLER

Aloe Juice Detangler

Ingredients

6 ½ -7 ounces of Aloe Vera Juice

8 ounce Spray Bottle

3-5 drops Lemon, vanilla or sweet orange essential Oils (for fragrance), if desired

1 tablespoon of Jojoba Oil

1 tablespoon of Avocado Oil

Instructions

1. Combine aloe vera juice and the oils together in a small mixing bowl.

2. Stir together until well combined.

3. Transfer aloe juice/oil mixture into a spray bottle.

4. Add few drops of the essential oil you are using.

5. Stir mixture to evenly distribute essential oil.

6. Store in a refrigerator.

7. Shake well before each use.

Natural Aloe Vera leave in & Detangler Mix

This recipe duals as a detangler and a leave-in. Before you condition or shampoo your hair, this detangler recipe is applied.

Ingredients

3 tbsps Aloe Vera juice

1 tbsp Grapeseed oil or any of your favorite essential oil

Instructions

1. Combine aloe vera juice and grapeseed oil together in a bowl.

2. Stir well until well combined.

3. Transfer into a spray bottle.

4. Shake bottle vigorously to combine mixture well.

5. Spray your hair with a rich portion of this detangler mix, until your hair is drenched.

NOTE: Breaking your hair into different sections may be of great help.

6. Rub in detangler mix with your hands into your hair, and smoothing your hair to make certain that each hair strand is richly coated.

7. Use comb or your fingers to detangle each parted hair sections.

8. Wash hair, pat dry and style as you would regularly.

CHAPTER FIVE- ORGANIC HAIR BUTTER TREATMENT

Rich Shea Hair Butter

Ingredients

shea butter

1 tbsp olive oil,

2 tsps almond oil,

1 tsp jamacian black castor oil,

1 tsp tea tree oil,

1 tbsp coconut oil,

1 tsp vitamin e oil.

Instructions

1. Transfer shea butter into a double boiler over medium low heat.

2. Melt until completely melted.

3. Take off from heat.

4. Measure in the olive oil, coconut oiil, almond oil, castor oil, vitamin E oil and tea tree oil.

5. Stir well until thoroughly combined.

NOTE: You can use an egg beater to whisk.

Hair Butter Moisturizer

Ingredients

Oil blend (flax seed oil, grape seed oil, olive oil, vegei oil, jojoba oil, fish oil, coconut oil,

tea tree oil or castor oil)

8 oz. Unrefined or Raw shea butter

Instructions

1. Combine shea butter and oils together in a large mixing bowl.

NOTE: If you are using more than 6 of the oils above; use a teaspoon each for the oil blend. If you are using less than 6 of them, you will use a tablespoon of each oil for the oil blend.

2. Transfer mixture into an electric mixer.

3. Mix until a smooth consistency is reached.

4. Transfer into a well covered container.

5. Store in a cool dry place.

Complete Hair Butter

Ingredients

10 drops of your favorite essential oil

8 ounce of unrefined organic Shea Butter

1 tablespoon of 100 percent Jojoba oil

Instructions

1. Combine jojoba oil and shea butter together in a small mixing bowl.

2. Mix with a hand mixer until well blended.

3. Measure in the essential oil.

4. Stir to distribute evenly into the mixture.

5. Transfer mixture into an airtight container

7. Apply as a sealant for your kinks and curls.

Tropical Aloe Hair Cream

Ingredients

2 heaping tbsps unrefined mango

Illipe butter

3 tbsps Tamanu oil

3 tbsps Organic Aloe Vera Juice

Shea butter

3 tbsps unrefined coconut oil

3 tbsps rosehip seed oil

8 tbsps Organic aloe Vera gel

3 tbsps olive oil

3-6 drops Vitamin E oil, unrefined

6-9 drops Tea tree oil

Instructions

1. Combine unrefined mango, illipe and shea butter together.

2. Mix well until well combined.

3. Transfer into a microwave until melted to liquid form.

4. Measure in the oils, aloe juice, aloe gel (every remaining ingredient)

5. Using a hand mixer, mix mixture until a fine creamy consistency is reached.

6. Keep in a refrigerator after application.

TIP: It can also be used as a body cream.

Hair Butter Mask with Pumpkin Seed

Ingredients

4 tablespoons pumpkin seed butter, organic

4 tablespoons extra dark Jamaican black castor oil

4 tablespoon of glycogen protein balancing conditioner

Instructions

1. Combine all ingredients together in a small mixing bowl.

2. Mix well until well combined.

3. Apply butter mask into the hair and hair strands.

4. Wear a plastic cap after application, for 60 minutes.

5. Wash off with and pat dry.

NOTE: This mask can also be used as a deep conditioner and as a detangler.

If you use as a detangler, make sure you rinse out with a hair conditioner of your choice and make sure every of the mask is removed from your hair.

Cocoa Butter Hair Balm

Ingredients

1/8 cup of Saffron Oil

1 ounce or 1 stick of Cocoa Butter

3 Tablespoons of Shea Butter

1/8 - ¼ cup of Olive Oil

3 Tablespoons of Coconut oil

Instructions

1. Combine shea butter, coconut oil and cocoa butter together in a mixing bowl.

2. Mix well until very combined.

3. Transfer into a double boiler and melt over low heat until completely melted.

4. Measure in saffron and olive oil and stir.

5. Transfer into a glass jar or container, cover and refrigerate.

NOTE: This product is semi-hardened at room temperature and it dissolves easily in the palms of your hand when you want to use.

TIP: You can apply this product after using leave-in condition, and before applying any curl defining product. This moisturizes the tips of the hair and the scalp.

Hair Butter Mask

Ingredients

1 teaspoon of pure cocoa powder

2 tablespoons of melted cocoa butter

1 tablespoons of olive oil

2 tablespoons of vegetable shortening

Instructions

1. Combine cocoa powder, melted cocoa butter, olive oil and vegetable shortening together in a mixing bowl.

2. Stir well until a fine and smooth consistency is reached.

3. Apply and rub on your hair edges and hair ends.

4. Take hair out of the way by pinning it up.

5. Leave mask on for 15-30 minutes.

6. Follow with shampoo and conditioner.

CHAPTER SIX - ORGANIC HAIR OIL TREATMENT

DIY Apricot Hair oil

This hair oil work well for twists and braids.

Ingredients

1oz. coconut oil

2 oz. apricot oil

1 oz. jojoba oil

1 tbsp avocado oil

1 tbsp safflower oil.

Instructions

1. Combine coconut oil, apricot oil, jojoba oil, avocado and safflower oil together in a mixing bowl.

2. Stir well to combine until a smooth consistency is reached.

3. Apply by massaging a rich amount of hair oil into your hair.

DIY Olive/Coconut Hair Oil Mix

Ingredients

4 ounce of coconut oil

3 ounce of olive oil

Instructions

1. Combine coconut oil and olive oil together in a small mixing bowl.

2. Stir well to combine.

3. Transfer into a bottle with a good cover.

4. Apply four times weekly.

DIY Castor Hair Oil

Ingredients

2 oz bottle

1 oz Jamaican Black Castor Oil

Essential oil for fragrance, if desired

2 tbsps grapeseed Oil

Instructions

1. Add 1 fluid ounce of castor oil into a 2 ounce bottle.

2. Measure in grapeseed oil and the essential oils together.

3. Cover bottle and shake vigorously.

4. Apply as you would any regular hair oil.

Hot Coconut Oil Hair Treat

Ingredients

1 tablespoons of Castor Oil

2 tablespoons of Coconut Oil

1 tablespoon of Jojoba Oil

2 drops of Vitamin E Oil

1 teaspoon of Peppermint Oil

Olive oil, optional

Instructions

1. Combine all the oils together in a small bowl.

2. Stir until well combined.

3. Transfer into a double boiler and melt over low heat until completely melted.

4. Allow oils to cool slightly but not lukewarm.

5. Apply to sectioned hair, from hair ends to the root and scalp.

6. Leave on, wearing plastic cap for 10-15 minutes.

7. Condition hair.

Egg Oil Hair Mask

Ingredients

2 eggs, beaten

5 tbsps of olive oil

Instructions

1. Combine eggs and olive oil together in a small mixing bowl.

2. Mix thoroughly until well combined and a smooth creamy consistency is reached.

3. Apply by massaging into your hair.

4. Leave on and cover hair with a plastic cap for 15 minutes.

5. Wash off and pat hair dry.

Hair Growth Oil Inversion

Ingredients

2-3 tbsps coconut oil or olive oil

Instructions

1. Measure in your scalp oil of choice into a microwavable bowl.

2. Warm for few minutes until lukewarm.

3. Bending over, facing down completely for 5 minutes; massage oil into your scalp with your hands.

TIP: The bending down inversion reverses blood flowing to the scalp and results in making your hair grow.

NOTE: If you are light headed, dizzy, sick or pregnant, do not do this.

4. Apply oil inversion for 7 days.

Hair Oil Mask

Ingredients

4 tablespoons of olive oil

2 whole eggs

Instructions

1. Combine eggs and olive oil together in a small mixing bowl.

2. Mix thoroughly until well combined and a smooth creamy consistency is reached.

3. Apply by massaging into your hair.

4. Leave on and cover hair with a plastic cap for 10 minutes.

5. Wash off and pat hair dry.

Carrier Oil Herbal Hair Treat

Ingredients

1 cup organic carrier oil

3-5 tbsps of herbs of your choice

Instructions

1. Infuse oils for 2 weeks by measuring herbs into oil mixture in a jar.

2. Stir well to combine and cover well.

3. Set aside for 2 weeks until flavors have been released and the oil infused.

TIP: Shake jar vigorously on a daily basis.

4. Strain out herbs using a mesh strainer or cheesecloth.

5. Transfer herbal infused oil into a jar or container.

6. Store in a refrigerator.

NOTE: Herbal hair oil will keep for 6 months if well refrigerated.

Hair Length Oil Mix

Ingredients

3 drops cedarwood essential oil

1/8 cup jojoba oil

3 drops lemon essential oil

1/8 cup grapeseed oil

3 drops rosemary essential oil

3 drops lavender essential oil

3 drops thyme essential oil

Instructions

1. Combine jojoba oil, grapeseed oil, and all the essential oils together in a small mixing bowl.

2. Stir well to combine.

3. Apply by using your hands to massage oil mix into your scalp.

TIP: Focus hair oil mix on the affected hair loss areas.

4. Store in a dark, cool and dry place.

NOTE: Do not use rosemary essential oil if you are heavy with child.

Hot Oil Treatment for Hair Growth

Ingredients

3 drops thyme essential oil

1/8 cup jojoba oil

3 drops lavender essential oil

3 drops rosemary essential oil

1/8 cup grapeseed oil

3 drops cedarwood essential oil

Instructions

1. Combine all oils and essential oils together.

2. Stir to combine until well mixed.

3. Apply by massaging into your scalp at night.

TIP: Focus on thinning areas.

4. Wash off and pat hair dry in the morning.

Organic DIY Hot Hair Oil Treat

Ingredients

Castor Oil

Olive Oil

Instructions

1. Combine castor and olive oil together in a mixing bowl.

2. Stir well to combine.

3. Transfer into a pot and heat over medium high heat.

4. Heat until warm. Take off from heat once warm.

5. Apply to the ends of your hair to your hair root and scalp.

TIP: Organic hot hair oil treat can be used before you wash hair

6. Leave on for 60 minutes or more.

Beautiful Hair Oil

Ingredients

1 teaspoon of neem oil, if desired

1 tablespoon of castor oil

1 tablespoon of organic argan oil

Few of drops essential oils, if desired

1 tablespoon of coconut oil

1 tablespoon of olive oil

1 tablespoon of broccoli seed oil

Instructions

1. Combine neem oil, castor oil, argan oil, coconut oil, olive oil and broccoli seed oil together in a mixing bowl.

2. Stir well to combine.

TIP: You can warm the oil mixture if you like.

3. Measure in essential oils drop.

4. Stir well to incorporate.

5. Wash hair well, clean and dry well.

6. Apply to your hair and scalp by massaging with your hands.

7. Cover your hair with a plastic cap and leave mixture in hair over the night.

8. Use clarifying shampoo to wash oil mixture out of your hair and scalp; and pat dry.

TIP: Tweak ingredients to get an increase in quantity of recipe.

9. Style and condition your hair.

NOTE: Treat hair with this beautiful hair oil treat.

Hair Power Oil

Ingredients

½ large bottle of Cayenne Pepper

45 cut tea bags

2-4 drops onion seed oil

30 Biotin pills, blended

1-2 drops garlic seed oil

Instructions

1. Combine cayenne pepper, tea bags and biotin pills together in a mixing bowl.

2. Stir to combine.

3. Infuse in an oven for 5 hours.

4. Take off from heat and set aside to cool to room temperature.

5. Stirring occasionally.

6. Use cheesecloth or mesh strainer to strain out the tea from the oil.

7. Measure in onion and garlic oil into the tea infused mixture.

8. Store in a dark, cool and dry place.

CHAPTER SEVEN - ORGANIC HAIR GROWTH TREATMENT

Mustard Hair Growth Mask

Ingredients

2 tablespoons olive oil

2 tablespoons ground mustard powder

1 egg yolk

2 teaspoons sugar

2 tablespoons hot water

Instructions

1. Combine mustard, water, egg yolk, sugar and oil together in a small mixing bowl.

2. Stir well until a smooth consistency is reached.

3. Apply to sectioned hair, massage hair growth mask into the scalp.

NOTE: Do not put to hair tips or hair ends.

4. Cover your hair with a plastic wrap or cap.

TIP: Place a hot damp towel on the plastic wrap to keep heat in. It will start burning quite fast, but its a good one.

If you feel the burning might be an allergy, wash off immediately.

5. Leave on for 15-60 minutes.

6. Wash off completely with warm water and pat hair dry.

7. Apply shampoo.

NOTE: Use hair growth mask twice weekly for 4-8 weeks, for maximum results.

Essential Blend Growth Oil

Ingredients

½ teaspoon jojoba oil

3 drops lavender

2 drops rosemary

2 drops thyme

4 teaspoon grapeseed oil

Instructions

1. Combine jojoba oil, grapeseed oil and the essential oils together in an applicator/spray bottle.

2. Shake vigorously to combine.

3. Apply by massaging into the scalp for 2 minutes.

4. Cover hair with a warm damp towel.

5. Leave on for 60 minutes.

6. Wash hair out with a mild shampoo and pat dry.

TIP: Use daily for 28 weeks.

Hair Force Deep Conditioner

HFDC contains a hygroscopic substance that keeps hair moist. This recipe adds protein to your hair and in turn grows your hair and strengthens it.

Ingredients

5 drops peppermint oil

1/4 Cup olive oil

1 egg, beaten

1/8 Cup honey

1 avocado

1 teaspoon of biotin powder

Instructions

1. Combine peppermint oil, olive oil, beaten egg, honey, avocado and biotin powder together.

2. Mix to combine, until a batter-like consistency is reached.

3. Make sure hair is damp.

4. Apply a rich layer to your hair.

5. Cover your hair with a plastic cap or wrap for 30-60 minutes.

6. Wash off and pat hair dry.

Rich Herbal Infused Growth Serum

Ingredients

1 cup of distilled water

10 drops of Lavender Essential Oil

2 tbsps of Dried Nettle Leaf

10 drops of Rosemary Essential Oil

2 tbsps of Natural Aloe Vera Gel

10 drops of Clary Sage Essential Oil

2 tbsps of Horsetail Leaf (if desired)

Instructions

1. Bring distilled water to a boil.

2. Toss in horsetail and dried nettle leaf.

3. Set aside until the water becomes cool.

4. Using a mesh strainer or cheesecloth, strain out the leaves.

5. Transfer liquid into a spray bottle.

6. Measure in lavender, rosemary, clary sage essential oils and aloe vera gel into the spray bottle.

7. Shake vigorously to evenly distribute.

8. Transfer bottle into a refrigerator for 3 months.

TIP: Leave stored in the refrigerator, 3 months before usage.

9. Shake well before each use; apply by spraying richly on your hair roots, 1-2 times daily.

Hair Health Growth mixture

Ingredients

2 avacados

1-2 bananas (depends on hair length)

2 teaspoons shea butter

2 to 3 drops tea tree oil

1 drop eucalyptus oil

Instructions

1. Combine Avocado, banana and shea butter into an electric blender or food processor.

2. Blend until a smooth consistency is reached.

3. Transfer into a bowl and measure in tea tree oil and eucalyptus oil.

4. Stir well to evenly distribute.

5. Apply by using your hands to massage into your scalp and your hair.

6. Use a wide tooth comb to comb hair.

7. Leave on for 5-10 minutes.

8. Wash off and pat hair dry.

Hair Smoothie from the Caribbean

This potion leaves your hair silky, soft, smooth, strong and healthy.

Ingredients

½ avocado (ripe)

½ cup of Coconut milk

½ banana (ripe)

1 tablespoon of Castor oil

2 tablespoon of Rosemary

1 teaspoon of Cayenne Pepper

Instructions

1. Combine avocado, coconut milk, banana, castor oil, rosemary and cayenne pepper together.

2. Stir together and transfer into an electric blender.

3. Blend until a smooth consistency is reached.

4. Apply mixture to the tip of your hair, along your hair strands and down to the root and scalp.

5. Leave on for 15-60 minutes.

6. Wash off with warm water and pat hair dry.

TIP: ingredients can be tweaked, depending on the length of hair.

Apple Cider Vinegar Growth Rinse

Ingredients

2 tablespoons rosemary dried leaf

1 cup apple cider vinegar

1 cup water

Instructions

1. Measure vinegar into a small mixing bowl.

2. Add in rosemary into the mixing bowl.

3. Stir to combine and transfer into the microwave for 30 seconds.

4. Strain vinegar.

TIP: Use the smallest available strainer.

5. Add water and stir well to combine.

6. Apply as you would a regular rinse.

DIY Organic Conditioner (Hair-Growth-Stimulator)

Ingredients

¼ cup of plain natural yogurt

1 egg

1 teaspoon of fresh lemon juice

8 to 10 drops of eucalyptus oil (or olive oil, or rosemary oil, or rosemary/olive oil and canola oil)

Instructions

1. Combine yogurt, beaten egg and lemon juice together.

2. Stir to combine and transfer into an electric blender.

3. Blend until a smooth consistency is reached.

4. Apply massaging on your scalp and hair.

5. Leave on for 20-30 minutes.

6. Wash off your hair and pat dry.

DIY Coconut/Honey Cooling Hair Mask

Ingredients

Castor oil

Avocado oil

10-20 drops peppermint essential oil

Olive oil

Raw honey

Shea moisture deep conditioning mask

Organic Coconut Milk

Instructions

1. Combine castor, olive, avocado oils and honey together in a bowl.

2. Stir well until well combined.

3. Mix in the deep conditioning mask and coconut milk together into the castor/honey mixture.

4. Stir well until a smooth, thick and creamy consistency is reached.

5. Measure in peppermint essential oil.

6. Stir well to incorporate essential oil into the mixture.

7. Wash hair and pat dry.

8. Apply cooling hair mask to damp hair.

9. Leave on for 30 minutes.

10. Wash off and pat hair dry.

CHAPTER EIGHT- ORGANIC HAIR GEL TREATMENT

Organic Aloe Hair Gel

Ingredients

3 egg whites

1-2 tablespoons vegetable glycerin

2/3 cup aloe Vera gel

5-8 drops essential oil(s) of choice (orange and vanilla extract)

1/8 cup of water

Instructions

1. Combine egg whites, vegetable glycerin, aloe gel and water together in a small mixing bowl.

2. Transfer aloe gel mixture into an electric blender.

3. Blend for 20 seconds, until a smooth consistency is reached.

4. Transfer into a container and cover well.

5. Store in a refrigerator until you want to apply.

Aloe Pectin Hair Jelly

Ingredients

1 cup aloe vera juice

1 (approx. 1.60 oz.) packet instant fruit pectin

¼ teaspoons honey

¼ teaspoons agave nectar

2 teaspoon EVOO

1 teaspoon sweet almond oil

5-7 drops of your favorite essential oils, (for fragrance), if desired

Instructions

1. Carefully and slowly add pectin in a stream into a mixing bowl.

NOTE: To avoid fruit pectin clumps, you need to make sure you are pouring slowly.

2. Stir in aloe vera juice.

3. Measure in agave nectar, honey, evoo and sweet almond oil.

4. Stir to combine until thoroughly mixed.

5. Measure in the essential oils.

6. Stir to again to evenly distribute essential oils into the aloe mixture.

7. Transfer aloe gel mixture into a bowl; cover very well.

8. Store in a refrigerator.

Chamomint Hair Styling Gel

Ingredients

1 tablespoon lemon juice

1/2 teaspoon xanthan gum powder

1 tablespoon/2 teabags of chamomile

1 cup water

½ tablespoon/1 teabag of mint

1/3 cup aloe vera juice

1 teaspoon maple syrup

Instructions

1. Bring cup of water to a boil.

2. Measure in chamomile and mint into boiling water.

3. Set aside to release tea flavors into the liquid and cool to room temperature.

4. Using a mesh strainer, tea strainer, or cheesecloth, strain out the tea from the liquid and discard teabags.

5. Measure in lemon juice, xanthan gum powder, aloe vera juice and maple syrup into the herbal tea.

6. Whisk all ingredients together.

7. Set aside to rest for a minute.

NOTE: Xanthan gum will thicken gradually.

TIP: Add a little more xanthan gum if your desired degree of thickness has not been reached, and add a little more water if it turns out too thick.

Matilda's Organic Curls Cream

Ingredients

1 jar or tube of Non-Flaking Gel or Aloe

1 tablespoon avocado oil, coconut oil, olive oil, mango butter or jojoba oil

2 tablespoons of pure shea butter,

Instructions

1. Combine aloe or non flaking gel, avocado oil, and shea butter together.

2. Mix well until a smooth consistency is reached.

3. Wash hair and apply by massaging cream into your scalp and hair with your hands.

4. Use a wide tooth brush to comb hair in, and to form definition.

5. Shake your hair and you are good.

Styling Cream Moisturizer

Ingredients

6 tbsps your favorite moisturizing conditioner

12 tbsps aloe vera gel

2 pinches cinnamon

½ tsp your favorite oil (you can use evoo)

2 tsps blue agave nectar

Tea tree or jasmine essential oils

Instructions

1. Combine your moisturizing conditioner, aloe vera gel, cinnamon, evoo oil and blue agave nectar together in a small bowl.

2. Stir thoroughly to combine until a thick consistency is reached.

TIP: The end result should be light when compared to a gel, but should have a thicker consistency than an average styling cream.

3. Transfer mixture into a glass jar.

Hair Refreshing Styling Spray

Ingredients

2 teaspoons Epsom salt

1 cup hot water

1/3 cup aloe vera gel

1 tablespoon jojoba or olive Oil

2 tablespoons Conditioner

Instructions

1. Combine epsom salt, water, aloe vera gel, jojoba oil and conditioner together.

2. Stir to combine.

3. Transfer into a spray bottle.

4. Shake vigorously before use.

5. Store in a refrigerator.

6. a) Wash hair.

b) Apply by spraying on damp hair to style.

7. Apply by spraying on dry hair to revive and refresh the hair in the afternoon

TIP: In hot temperatures, do not use oil for this recipe; substitute with a bit of honey and/or aloe vera juice as a substitute.

NOTE: You can experiment and tweak ingredients to suit your hair type. The effectiveness of this hair styling spray depends on the brands of the products used.

Glowing Waves Coconut Milk/Oil Conditioner

This recipe is a conditioner that helps to moisturize your curls. Works well for all hair type, gives your hair, strength; and gives an out of this world kinda glow. It remedies hair loss and stimulates hair growth.

Ingredients

1 tablespoon your favorite hair conditioner

1 tablespoon cane molasses

3 tablespoon coconut milk (or add to taste)

1 tablespoon coconut oil

1 tablespoon honey

1 tablespoon rosemary infused olive oil

Instructions

1. In a small bowl, combine your favorite hair conditioner, cane molasses, coconut milk, coconut oil, honey and rosemary infused olive oil together.

2. Stir to combine, until thoroughly combined.

3. Shampoo hair 3 days before applying hair mixture.

4. Apply mixture by massaging from your hair tips to the roots and scalp.

5. Leave on for 60 minutes or more.

NOTE: You can substitute the olive oil for any other oil of your choice.

DIY Leave-In Conditioner

This recipe fights against hair loss, dandruff, dry and itchy scalp, and it promotes hair growth.

Ingredients

10 small squirts of Lime Juice

½ cup of Aloe Juice and gel

1 cup distilled water

Milk/Water from 1 coconut

1 tablespoon of melted Shea butter

1 tablespoon of melted Coconut Oil

1 teaspoon of Olive oil

½ teaspoon of Thyme oil

1 teaspoon of Rosemary oil

Instructions

1. Combine lime juice, aloe gel & juice, distilled water, coconut milk, melted shea butter, melted coconut oil, olive oil, thyme oil and rosemary oil together in a small bowl.

2. Mix until a smooth consistency is reached.

3. Transfer leave -in conditioner into a spray bottle.

4. Apply as you would a regular leave-in conditioner.

Protein Filled Mud mask

This recipe grows and strengthens your hair, brings hair back into form and gives time trusted elasticity

Ingredients

1 cup aloe vera juice/coconut milk

2 cups Nupur henna mixture (see below)

Your favorite moisture rinse out conditioner

1 large egg, beaten

2 1/2 tbsps coconut oil

4 tbsps agave nectar/honey

Instructions

1. Combine ayurvedic henna mixture with coconut milk or aloe vera juice together in a bowl.

2. Stir well until well combined.

3. Measure in the coconut oil, beaten egg and the moisture rinse out conditioner.

4. Stir well to evenly distribute.

5. Apply by massaging into your hair ends, hair strands, hair roots and scalp.

6. Leave on for 60-180 minutes.

7. Cover hair with a plastic cap or wrap

8. Wash off with water and a protein-free, rich in moisture conditioner.

TIP: This gives your hair a glowing and popping feel.

NOTE: a) Avoid bending, much movement that may affect the position of your hair while the mud mask is still in your hair. This prevents hair from knotting and tangling. b) Ayurvedic henna mixture (Brahmi, hibiscus powder, shikakai, aloe vera,

amla, bhringraj, neem, and jatamansi powders).

CHAPTER NINE- NATURAL SHAVING CREAM TREATMENT

Homemade Shaving Cream

This shaving cream makes your skin luxuriantly pampered with this recipe. It's a great alternative for those with skins that are sensitive.

Ingredients

4 tablespoons solid shea butter

3 tablespoons coconut oil

2 tablespoons sweet almond oil

10-12 drops pure lavender essential oil, if desired

Instructions

1. Mix coconut oil and shea butter together

2. Transfer into a double boiler over very low heat and melt.

3. Stir from time to time. Take mixture off heat once mixture has melts totally.

4. Measure in lavender oil and almond and stir to incorporate oils well.

5. Pour mixture into a bowl and refrigerate to allow mixture solidify.

6. Whip shaving cream mixture using an electric mixer or a stand mixer.

7. Set whipped mixture aside before you transfer in a well covered jar or container.

TIP: Do not use beyond a month.

DIY Shaving Cream

Ingredients

Makes: 2 cups

1/2 (4 ounce) cup of coconut oil

1/4 cup olive oil

1/2 (4 ounce) cup shea butter

20-25 drops eucalyptus essential oil

Instructions

1. Combine shea butter and coconut oil in a mixing bowl.

2. Transfer bowl mixture into a double boiler over medium low heat and melt.

3. Once melted, take off from heat and transfer to a bowl.

4. Measure olive oil into the mixture and stir to incorporate.

5. Refrigerate until mixture solidifies.

6. Remove from the refrigerator.

7. Using a hand mixer or standing mixer, whip bowl's mixture until stiff peaks are formed, for 3 minutes.

8. Meanwhile, as you whip mixture, measure in the essential oils.

9. Transfer whipped shaving cream into a well covered jar and store.

CHAPTER TEN - COCONUT OIL RECIPES FOR HAIR TREATMENT

The ultimate shine product, coconut oil! This organic all-in-one hair care product is loaded with lauric acid, anti-microbial properties, and medium chain fatty acids that gives hair strength, grows your hair and conditions your scalp. Coconut oil is loaded with minerals, vitamins and many other nourishments, nutrients and benefits for your hair.

Coconut Oil Hair Conditioner

Ingredient

1/4 tsp coconut oil, warmed (for thinner, shorter hair), 1/2 tsp coconut oil (for thicker, longer hair)

Instructions

1. Warm coconut oil.

2. Transfer into the palm of your hands.

3. Apply to hair shaft and hair ends, smoothing with your hands.

TIP: For a damaged or dry hair, measure 3-4 drops of geranium and/or sandalwood essential oils.

They serve as a leave-in and deep conditioners.

Coconut Oil Scalp Conditioner and Hair Growth Serum

Ingredients

1 tsp coconut oil

Instructions

1. Apply by massaging on the scalp using your hands as you massage, pressing gently.

2. Continue massage for 10 minutes.

TIP: Apply 3-4 times weekly.

Coconut Oil Anti-Dandruff

Ingredients

5 drops lavender, thyme, wintergreen or tea tree essential oils

2 tsps coconut oil

Instructions

1. Combine coconut oil and one of the essential oils above into a small bowl.

2. Stir until well blended.

3. Apply by massaging well into your scalp; cover your whole scalp-hair area.

4. Leave on, covering with a plastic cap and stay in the sun for 20-30 minutes.

TIP: This increases heat, or use a hand dryer.

Coconut Oil Frizz Tame

Ingredients

1/4-1 tsp coconut oil (depends on hair length)

Instructions

1. Warm oil.

2. Pour into the palm of your hands.

3. Apply by smoothing oil from hair ends to hair roots.

4. Use a hand dryer to blow dry your hair.

TIP: Can be used as a detangler, note, and use a little if you have short and thin hair. You can also leave the oil on to act as a sunscreen for your hair.

Coconut Oil Lice Prevention & Cure Leave-in Conditioner

Ingredients

3 tbsps coconut oil

1 tsp ylang ylang oil

1 tsp tea tree oil

1 tsp anise oil

1 cup distilled water

2 cups apple cider vinegar

Instructions

TIP: Double recipe for a fuller, longer hair (hair passing the shoulder).

1. Combine first four ingredients together in a small mixing bowl.

2. Apply by massaging oils over the entire scalp and hair area on your head.

3. Work through your hair with a comb or your fingers.

4. Leave on for 120 minutes.

5. Cover hair with a plastic cap.

TIP: Use hair dryer or stay under the sun for heat.

6. After waiting time, comb hair.

7. Wash hair well and pat dry.

8. Combine water and vinegar into a spray bottle.

9. Shake vigorously to mix.

10. Apply to hair as you rub in gently into your hair

11 Rinse hair one more time and comb.

12. Apply light coconut oil to hair, cover with a plastic cap and style your hair.

TIP: Leave on till you wash your hair again

Coconut Oil Hair Shampoo

Ingredients

1 cup liquid castile soap

1/3 cup coconut oil

1/3 cup coconut milk

50-60 drops essential oils (lavender, peppermint, wild orange, lemon grass, clary sage and rosemary)

Instructions

1. Combine coconut milk and coconut oil together.

2. Stir well until combined.

3. Warm over very super low heat.

NOTE: If heat is too high, nutrients in the mixture would be destroyed.

4. Transfer into a container.

5. Measure in castile soap and shake bottle vigorously.

6. Measure in the essential oil(s).

7. Shake bottle to incorporate.

8. Cover well.

9. Apply by squeezing on hair as you wash hair and rinse out well.

Coconut Oil Hair Conditioner

Ingredients

2/3 cup coconut oil

1 tbsp Jojoba oil

1 tbsp vitamin E oil

10 drops of your favorite essential oil

Instructions

1. Combine coconut oil, jojoba oil, vitamin E oil and any of your favorite essential oil in a mixing bowl.

2. Mix well to combine, using a hand mixer until a creamy and smooth consistency is reached.

3. After shampooing, apply 1-2 tsps of the coconut oil conditioner to hair and smooth through your hair.

4. Wash off and pay hair dry

NOTE: If you use hair dyes, coconut oil will fade the hair dye, especially red hair tint. Other hair tints/dyes may not fade.

Coconut Oil Dark Hair Color Base

For darker hair color

Ingredients

2 tbsps coconut oil

1 tbsp spent grounds

1 cup strong coffee

Instructions

1. Combine all ingredients together in a small mixing bowl

2. Stir to combine well.

3. Apply by massaging into hair.

4. Leave on for 45-60 minutes.

5. Wash off, pat dry and style your hair as desired.

Coconut Oil Blonde Hair Color Base

Ingredients

1/2 cup strong chamomile tea

1/4 cup fresh lemon juice

1/4 cup coconut oil

Instructions

1. Combine all ingredients together in a small bowl.

2. Stir to combine and transfer into an electric blender.

3. Blend until mixture emulsifies.

4. Apply to you entire hair length, tip and roots.

5. Wear plastic cap and leave on for 45-75minutes.

TIP: For added heat, stay in the sun or use hair dryer for the duration of leave-on time.

CHAPTER ELEVEN - HAIR PAMPERING RECIPES

Scented Hair Aromatherapy Recipe

This recipe gives a lovely fragrance to your hair.

Ingredient

1 drop of Lavender/Rosemary/Sandalwood

Instructions

1. Choose any one of the essential oils listed in the ingredient list.

2. Apply 1 drop to the bristles of a hair brush.

3. Use hair brush to brush your hair thoroughly.

Dandruff Fighting Scalp Treatment

This recipe combats fungi and absorbs excessive moisture on the skin.

Ingredients

1-2 tsps salt.

Few drops of water

Instructions

1. Apply by sprinkling salt on your scalp.

2. Moisten your hands with water and massage scalp thoroughly with wet hands for 10-15 minutes.

3. Wash, pat dry your hair. Apply hair conditioning cream.

END

Thank you for reading my book. If you enjoyed it, won't you please take a moment to look at my other titles?

Thanks!

Matilda C Butler

www.ingramcontent.com/pod-product-compliance
Lightning Source LLC
Chambersburg PA
CBHW050400290526
45786CB00003B/1069